Behavioral Therapy

BEHAVIORL THERAPY

Behavioural Therapy Made Super Easy; Simple to Follow Steps That Enable you to Kill Anxiety, Depression, Stress, Trauma, and Post Traumatic Stress Disorder Part-1

BY
Tom Bhowey

Behavioral Therapy

Table of Contents

A Brief Background 12
Behavior Therapy Based on Classical Conditioning...........14
Behavior Therapy Based on Operant Conditioning........... 17
Behavior Therapy in Practice.......................................26
Goals of Behavior Therapy..26
The Role of the Therapist in Behavior Therapy................27
What does Behavior Therapy Treat?..............................28
ADHD and Behavior Therapy......................................31
How Behavior Therapy Works.....................................31
What to Expect From Behavior Therapy........................32
How Behavior Therapy Can Help Kids with ADHD........... 34
A.   Cognitive Behavioral Therapy...............................39
Uses for CBT..40
What happens during CBT sessions?............................41
Pros and cons of CBT...43
The Effectiveness of Cognitive Behavioral Therapy.........45
How Cognitive Behavioral Therapy Works....................45
Precautions to Take Before Starting Cognitive Behavioral Therapy..47
The History of Cognitive Behavioral Therapy.................48
Principles of Cognitive Behavioral Therapy...................53
Cognitive-Behavioral Therapy - The Basics...................57
What Constitutes Cognitive Behavioral Therapy?...........63

Behavioral Therapy

Cognitive Behavioral Therapy and the Treatment of Addiction...........68
How Can Cognitive-Behavioral Therapy Help OCD Sufferers?...........71
Cognitive Behavioral Therapy for Treating Autism...........73
Cognitive Behavioral Therapy for Anxiety - Does It Work? 76
Can Cognitive Behavioral Therapy Be Useful For Anger Management?...........79
Using Cognitive Behavior Therapy (CBT) for Panic Attacks...........82
A. Behavioral Activation Therapy...........84
Behavioral Therapy for Autism...........85
Behavioral Therapy to Cure Panic Disorder...........88
B. Aversion Therapy...........91
C. Cognitive-Behavioral Play Therapy...........91
D. System Desensitization...........92
Finding the Right Behavior Therapist...........97
How to Tell If Your Therapist Uses Cognitive Behavioral Therapy...........98

Behavioral Therapy

© Copyright 2021 - All rights reserved.

The content contained within this book may not be reproduced, duplicated or transmitted without direct written permission from the author or the publisher.

Under no circumstances will any blame or legal responsibility be held against the publisher, or author, for any damages, reparation, or monetary loss due to the information contained within this book. Either directly or indirectly.

Legal Notice:

This book is copyright protected. This book is only for personal use. You cannot amend, distribute, sell, use, quote or paraphrase any part, or the content within this book, without the consent of the author or publisher.

Disclaimer Notice:

Please note the information contained within this document is for educational and entertainment purposes only. All effort has been executed to present accurate, up to date, and reliable, complete information. No warranties of any kind are declared or implied. Readers acknowledge that the author is not engaging in the rendering of legal, financial, medical or professional advice. The content within this book has been derived from various sources. Please consult a licensed professional before attempting any techniques outlined in this book.

Behavioral Therapy

By reading this document, the reader agrees that under no circumstances is the author responsible for any losses, direct or indirect, which are incurred as a result of the use of information contained within this document, including, but not limited to, — errors, omissions, or inaccuracies.

Behavioral Therapy

Introduction

Behavioral therapy, or behavioral modification, is a psychological technique based on the premise that specific, observable, maladaptive, badly adjusted, or self-destructing behaviors can be modified by learning new, more appropriate behaviors to replace them.

Since its early 20th-century beginnings, behavioral therapy has prided itself above all on being scientific. So avoiding such unquantifiable as needs want, and motivation, together with excursions into the unconscious and transpersonal. Instead, it has concentrated on observing and analyzing behavioral and cognitive functioning, diagnosing unproductive ways of dealing with life and instituting systematic changes to improve outcomes. Therapists discuss methods and expectations with clients; the clients' participation is negotiated, and measures to monitor effectiveness are established. Techniques used are practical and direct, including those listed below. Counter Conditioning An undesirable response to a stimulus is replaced by one newly elicited. Desensitization The client is relaxed deeply, then gradually he or she is exposed to an anxiety -provoking situation. Aversion Conditioning A stimulus that is attractive to the client, but would lead to undesirable results, is paired with an unpleasant event to break the pattern. Role-Playing The therapist demonstrates more effective behaviors in the session. The client tries these out in real-life situations. Behavior Rehearsal The client copies the therapist's staged rehearsal of a forthcoming situation that is expected to be problematic.BenefitsBehavioral therapy can be a useful treatment tool in an array of mental illnesses and symptoms of mental illness that involve maladaptive behavior, such as substance abuse, aggressive behavior, anger management, eating disorders, phobias, and anxiety disorders. It is also used to treat organic disorders such as incontinence and insomnia by changing the behaviors that might be contributing to these disorders cognitive therapy this grew out of behavioral thinking in the 1960s and concentrates on how people's experiences are governed by their perceptions. For example, cognitive theory sees depression as the result of sad thinking, rather than believing conversely that sad thinking is the result of a state of depression. Cognitive Restructuring Transforming a client's thinking processes to influence behavior and emotions. Rational-emotive Approach Replacing irrational beliefs with rational ones. Assumption of Responsibility Getting clients to accept that no one else "makes" them think, feel, or do anything. Unlike traditional psychotherapy and many other forms of therapy, cognitive behavioral therapy does not involve lengthy time frames or extensive investigation into past life events. Cognitive ehavior therapy is a goal-oriented short-term process, predominantly focused upon the present and future. Most cognitive behavior therapy treatments range from a few weeks to a few months in duration. Cognitive behavior therapy therapists take an active role in the treatment process, and the patient is usually expected to complete types of "homework" exercises involving reinforcement of positive patterns. IndeedArticle Submission, these "corrective experiences" that occur outside of the therapy sessions are an important part of treatment.

In behavioral therapy, the goal is to reinforce desirable behaviors and eliminate unwanted or maladaptive ones. Behavioral therapy is rooted in the principles of behaviorism, a school of thought focused on the idea that we learn from our environment. The techniques used in this type of treatment are based on the theories of classical conditioning and operant conditioning.

One important thing to note about the various behavioral therapies is that unlike some other types of therapy that are rooted in insight (such as psychoanalytic and humanistic therapies), behavioral therapy is action-based. Behavioral therapists are focused on using the same learning strategies that led to the formation of unwanted behaviors.

Because of this, behavioral therapy tends to be highly focused. The behavior itself is the problem and the goal is to teach clients new behaviors to minimize or eliminate the issue. Old learning led to the development of a problem and so the idea is that new learning can fix it.

1.2　A Brief Background

Edward Thorndike was one of the first to refer to the idea of modifying behavior. Other early pioneers of behavior therapy included psychologists Joseph Wolpe and Hans Eysenck.

Behaviorist B.F. Skinner's work had a major influence on the development of behavior therapy and his work introduced many of the concepts and techniques that are still in use today.

Later on, psychologists such as Aaron Beck and Albert Ellis began adding a cognitive element to behavioral strategies to form a treatment approach known as cognitive-behavioral therapy (CBT).

The Foundation of Behavioral Therapy

In order to understand how behavioral therapy works, let's start by exploring the two basic principles that contribute to behavioral therapy: classical and operant conditioning.

Classical conditioning involves forming associations between stimuli. Previously neutral stimuli are paired with a stimulus that naturally and automatically evokes a response. After repeated pairings, an association is formed and the previously neutral stimulus will come to evoke the response on its own.

Operant conditioning focuses on how reinforcement and punishment can be utilized to either increase or decrease the frequency of a behavior. Behaviors followed by desirable consequences are more likely to occur again in the future, while those followed by negative consequences become less likely to occur.

Behavior Therapy Based on Classical Conditioning

Classical conditioning is one way to alter behavior, and several techniques exist that can produce such change. Originally known as behavior modification, this type of therapy is often referred to today as applied behavior analysis.

Some of the techniques and strategies used in this approach to therapy include:

1. Flooding

    This process involves exposing people to fear-invoking objects or situations intensely and rapidly. It is often used to treat phobias, anxiety and other stress-related disorders. During the process, the individual is prevented from escaping or avoiding the situation.

    For example, flooding might be used to help a client who is suffering from an intense fear of dogs. At first, the client might be exposed to a small friendly dog for an extended period during which he or she cannot leave. After repeated exposures to the dog during which nothing bad happens, the fear response begins to fade.

2. Systematic Desensitization

This technique involves having a client make a list of fears and then teaching the individual to relax while concentrating on these fears. The use of this process began with psychologist John B. Watson and his famous Little Albert experiment in which he conditioned a young child to fear a white rat. Later, Mary Cover Jones replicated Watson's results and utilized counterconditioning techniques to desensitize and eliminate the fear response.

Systematic desensitization is often used to treat phobias. The process follows three basic steps.

First, the client is taught relaxation techniques.

Next, the individual creates a ranked list of fear-invoking situations.

Starting with the least fear-inducing item and working their way up to the most fear-inducing item, the client confronts these fears under the guidance of the therapist while maintaining a relaxed state.

For example, an individual with a fear of the dark might start by looking at an image of a dark room before moving on to thinking about being in a dark room and then actually confronting his fear by sitting in a dark room. By pairing the old fear-producing stimulus with the newly learned relaxation behavior, the phobic response can be reduced or even eliminated.

3. Aversion Therapy

   This process involves pairing an undesirable behavior with an aversive stimulus in the hope that the unwanted behavior will eventually be reduced. For example, someone suffering from alcoholism might utilize a drug known as disulfiram, which causes severe symptoms such as headaches, nausea, anxiety, and vomiting when combined with alcohol. Because the person becomes extremely ill when they drink, the drinking behavior may be eliminated.

Behavior Therapy Based on Operant Conditioning

Many behavior techniques rely on the principles of operant conditioning, which means that they utilize reinforcement, punishment, shaping, modeling and related techniques to alter behavior. These methods have the benefit of being highly focused, which means that they can produce fast and effective results.

Some of the techniques and strategies used in this approach to behavioral therapy include:

1. Token Economies

    This type of behavioral strategy relies on reinforcement to modify behavior. Clients are allowed to earn tokens that can be exchanged for special privileges or desired items. Parents and teachers often use token economies to reinforce good behavior. Kids earn tokens for engaging in preferred behaviors and may even lose tokens for displaying undesirable behaviors. These tokens can then be traded for things such as candy, toys, or extra time playing with a favorite toy.

2. Contingency Management

This approach utilizes a formal written contract between the client and the therapist that outlines the behavior change goals, reinforcements, and rewards that will be given and the penalties for failing to meet the demands of the agreement. These types of agreements aren't just used by therapists—teachers and parents also often use them with students and children in the form of behavior contracts. Contingency contracts can be very effective in producing behavior changes since the rules are spelled out clearly in black-and-white, preventing both parties from backing down on their promises.

3. Modeling

This technique involves learning through observation and modeling the behavior of others. The process is based on Albert Bandura's social learning theory, which emphasizes the social components of the learning process. Rather than relying simply on reinforcement or punishment, modeling allows individuals to learn new skills or acceptable behaviors by watching someone else perform those desired skills. In some cases, the therapist might model the desired behavior. In other instances, watching peers engage in sought-after behaviors can also be helpful.

4. Extinction

Another way to produce behavior change is to stop reinforcing behavior in order to eliminate the response. Time-outs are a perfect example of the extinction process. During a time-out, a person is removed from a situation that provides reinforcement. For example, a child who starts yelling or striking other children would be removed from the play activity and required to sit quietly in a corner or another room where there are no opportunities for attention and reinforcement. By taking away the attention that the child found rewarding, unwanted behavior is eventually extinguished.

Behavioral Therapy

Chapter 1

What is Behavioral Therapy?

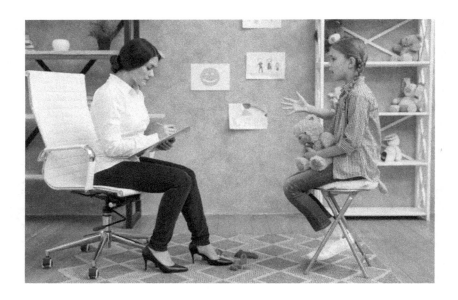

Behavioral therapy, also known as behavioral modification, is an approach to psychotherapy based on learning theory that aims to treat psychopathology through techniques that are designed to reinforce desired behaviors and eliminate undesired behaviors. Ancient philosophical traditions, such as Stoicism, provided the precursors of certain fundamental aspects of behavioral therapy. The

Behavioral Therapy

first occurrence of the term "behavioral therapy" may have been used in a 1953 research project by B.F. Skinner, Ogden Lindsley, Nathan H. Azrin, and Harry C. Solomon. Other early pioneers in this type of therapy include Joseph Wolpe and Hans Eysenck.

Behavioral therapy is considered to have three distinct points of origin: South Africa (Wolpe's group), the United States (Skinner), and the United Kingdom (Rachman and Eysenck). Eysenck, in particular, viewed behavioral problems as an interplay between environment, behavior, and personal characteristics. Skinner's group, on the other hand, took more of an operant conditioning approach, which involved a functional approach to assessment and interventions focused on contingency management (reward and punishment for positive and negative behavior, respectively, also known as the "token system") and behavioral activation.

Skinner became interested in individualizing programs to improve the learning of people with and without disabilities; he worked with Fred S. Keller to develop programmed instruction. Programmed instruction showed clinical success in treating aphasia rehabilitation. Skinner's student, Ogden Lindsley, is credited with forming a movement called "precision teaching," which developed a type of graphing program that kept track of how much progress the clients were making.

In the second half of the 20th century, many therapists began combining this therapy with the cognitive therapy of Aaron Beck and Albert Ellis, which created cognitive behavioral therapy. In some areas, the cognitive component added to the therapy (especially when it came to social phobia treatment), but in other areas, the cognitive component did not add to the therapy. This led to the pursuit of Third Generation Behavioral Therapies.

Third Generation Behavioral Therapies combines the basic principles of operant and respondent psychology with functional analysis and a Clinical formulation or case conceptualization of verbal behavior, which incorporates more of the view of the behavioral analysts. Some research shows that

Third Generation Behavioral Therapies are more effective in some cases than cognitive therapy, but more research needs to be done in order for the evidence to be conclusive.

Some of the most widely used approaches in behavioral therapy today include Acceptance and Commitment Therapy (ACT), Cognitive Behavioral Analysis System of

Psychotherapy (CBASP), behavioral activation (BA), and Integrative behavioral couples therapy. Behavioral therapy combines the principles of classical conditioning developed by Ivan Pavlov and the principles of operant conditioning developed by B. F. Skinner. There has been some confusion on how these two conditionings differ and how the various techniques of this have any common scientific basis. An online paper, "Reinforcing Behavioral Therapy, provides an answer to this confusion.

Operant conditioning has led to contingency management programs. These programs have been quite effective, even in adults who deal with schizophrenia. Respondent conditioning has led to systematic desensitization and exposure and response prevention. Social skills training teaches clients the skills to access reinforcers and to lessen life punishment. However, operant conditioning procedures in the meta-analysis had the greatest effect on training social skills. While social skills training had shown some effectiveness for schizophrenia, applying behavioral programs to schizophrenia has generally lost favor amongst many psychologists.

Behavioral therapy's core interventions are based on functional analysis. Amongst the many problems that behavioral therapy have functionally analyzed include intimacy in couples, forgiveness in couples, relationships, chronic pain, anorexia, depression, obesity, and anxiety. Functional analysis has even been applied to problems that therapists will often encounter with patients, including involuntary clients, partially engaged clients, and client resistance. This has led to considerable tools for therapists to use to enhance therapeutic effectiveness, including using positive reinforcement or operant conditioning.

This has led many to believe that behavioral therapy is as effective, if not more effective, to treating depression, attention-deficit hyperactivity disorder, and obsessive-compulsive disorder than drug treatment. Another successful form of therapy that has shown great success is Habit reversal training. This has proven highly effective in treating tics. The characteristics of behavioral therapy include being empirical (data-driven), contextual (focusing on environment and context), functional (interested in a behavior's consequence or effect), probabilistic (seeing behavior as statistically predictable), monistic (treating the person as a unit and rejecting mind-body dualism), and relational (analyzing bidirectional interactions).

Behavioral therapy developed from three different points of origin and has its roots in both operant conditioning and respondent conditioning. Behavioral therapy has proven to be as effective, if not more effective, than drug treatment when it comes to treating depression, attention-deficit hyperactivity disorder, and obsessive-compulsive disorder. Third Generation Behavioral Therapies that are widely used to great effect today originated from behavioral therapy. These are just some of the reasons why the discovery and development of behavioral therapy are so important in our world today.

Behavior Therapy in Practice

Behavior therapy begins with an in-depth assessment of the patient's condition including behavioral patterns. Patients may be required to answer questionnaires or keep daily journals so the therapist can recognize trends in behaviors, such as triggers of the behavior. Once the patient's condition is assessed, the patient and therapist agree on short and long-term goals for the therapy.

Goals of Behavior Therapy

The goals of behavior therapy are specific: to change or eliminate specific behavior. Typically, the therapist and the patient will work together to set clear goals for the course of therapy. However, patients do not always actively participate in their therapy. For example, people forced into behavior therapy (such as institutionalized patients or children by their parents) may be reluctant to participate at all.

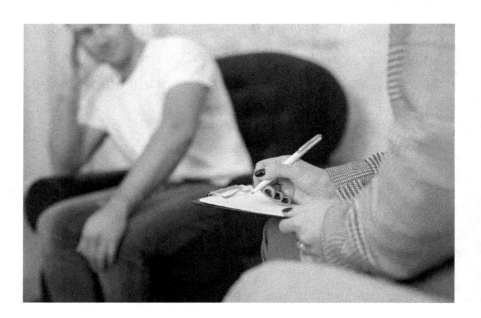

The Role of the Therapist in Behavior Therapy

A therapist may need to take on various roles throughout the course of behavior therapy. First, the therapist must be the "teacher" by helping the patient to recognize destructive behaviors and their patterns or triggers. Depending on the method of behavior therapy used, the therapist may act as a supportive person (such as when coping with stress caused from confronting a phobia) or as a harsh authority figure (such as when pushing a patient to deal with a phobia). A therapist may also work with family members to teach them skills for dealing with negative behaviors.

What does Behavior Therapy Treat?

Behavioral therapy can benefit people with a wide range of disorders. People most commonly seek behavioral therapy to treat:

- Depression
- Anxiety
- Panic disorders
- Anger issues

It can also help treat conditions and disorders such as:

- Eating disorders
- Post-traumatic stress disorder (PTSD)
- Bipolar disorder
- ADHD
- Phobias, including social phobias
- Obsessive-compulsive disorder (OCD)
- Self-harm
- Substance abuse

This type of therapy can benefit adults and children.

Behavior therapy is most commonly used for treating disorders in which the symptoms themselves are the problem. For example, some patients with a debilitating specific phobia may not present any other psychological symptoms. Symptom-based conditions, including obsessive-compulsive disorder, anxiety disorders, and impulse control disorders, have shown very responsive to behavior therapy.

Behavior therapy can also be used for disorders which are not necessarily symptom-based. For example, behavior therapy has proven effective in treating depression in some cases. One expert, Peter Lewinsohn, theorized that depression is actually a low rate of behavior which causes all

Behavioral Therapy

of the other symptoms. While this theory has been criticized and unaccepted by the psychological community, evidence shows that behavior therapy can treat depression. For depression,

treatment may be much more complex and involve the patient identifying certain trends in emotions and finding ways to avoid or overcome them through positive reinforcement. However, it is much more common for non-symptoms based psychological disorders to be treated with other approaches or a combination of cognitive and behavioral therapy.

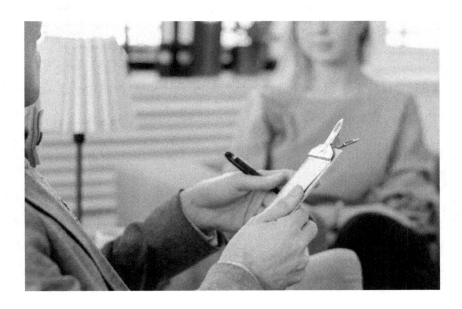

ADHD and Behavior Therapy

At a Glance;

- Behavior therapy focuses on replacing negative habits and actions with positive ones.
- Parents use a rewards system that targets very specific behaviors.
- Part of behavior therapy for ADHD is teaching parents how to change their behavior, too.

If your child has ADHD, you might be looking into treatment options. One non-medication approach that can be helpful for some kids is behavior therapy for ADHD. The goal of behavior therapy is to replace a child's negative actions and habits with positive ones. And parents are the ones who lead the process.

How Behavior Therapy Works

When some people hear the term therapy, they may think of clients sitting with a therapist to talk about emotions and work through problems. Behavior therapy is very different from this, however. It focuses on a person's actions, not on thoughts and emotions.

Therapists—typically clinical psychologists—work with clients to create a plan to help change behavior. The plan is designed to replace negative habits and actions with positive ones.

Behavior therapy for kids is as much about changing the parents' behavior as the child's. Parents can get into the habit of nagging and yelling, which can reinforce their child's negative actions. A big piece of behavior therapy is coaching parents on how to replace their negative actions with positive ones, too.

What to Expect From Behavior Therapy

So what can you expect from behavior therapy for ADHD? It starts with you, your child and the therapist having a meeting.

Together, you'll talk about the behaviors that are most challenging at school or home. Those might be things like talking out of turn, not finishing homework, or having angry outbursts.

The therapist will help you come up with a plan for you and your child to follow that addresses the most troublesome behaviors. The plans are based on a system of rewards and consequences. (That's why it's important for your child to be there. You'll need his help to come up with rewards that are really motivating!)

Next, you'll create a chart listing the specific actions your child needs to take. These should be clear, concrete and measurable, so your child knows exactly what the expectations are.

The chart can use pictures or words—or both. It should be posted at home where he can easily see and use it. When your child does what he's supposed to do, you'll check it off. And he'll earn points toward a reward.

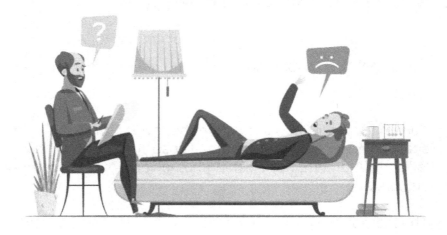

Once you start using the chart, you'll meet with the psychologist every week—without your child. The purpose of those sessions is to talk about how things are going, troubleshoot problems, and adjust the plan as needed. In essence, the therapist will be training you to be the "therapist" at home. Once a month, your child will join you at those sessions.

How Behavior Therapy Can Help Kids with ADHD

Behavior therapy can be helpful for lots of kids, and adults, too. But it can be especially helpful for kids with ADHD. Kids with ADHD can struggle with self-control and anger, which can lead to problem behaviors. It's also not uncommon for kids with ADHD to lie frequently about everyday tasks like chores.

Behavior therapy takes a very businesslike approach to help kids with ADHD change how they act and respond to situations. One of the goals is to eliminate arguing at home and give kids the motivation to change without parents being so involved.

The point of behavior therapy is to replace negative behaviors with positive ones. So the system of rewards and consequences is very specific. But whatever the reward is, it's always coupled with praise to reinforce good behavior. (Your child's teacher must be aware of this plan, so she can reinforce the behavior at school, too.)

Let's say one of the behaviors you want to change is putting off starting homework. On his chart, you'll put the desired behavior: "Start my homework when I'm supposed to."

You'll also decide on a reward. It might be: "For every five times I start on time, I'll get an extra hour of screen time." So each time he does his homework with only one cue from you, you'll mark it off and he'll earn points.

Equally important is the verbal recognition and praise he'll get from you. For instance, you might say, "You did a great job remembering to raise your hand in class. I'm really pleased with how hard you're trying."

If he doesn't remember to raise his hand, he simply doesn't get a point. But he doesn't get in trouble either or lose any points. The point is to reward positive behavior and ignore negative behavior.

If this approach isn't successful, however, you might need to switch to negative consequences like losing points. And if the negative behavior you're trying to change is aggression, you might have to use negative consequences in that situation, too.

Behavioral Therapy

Sometimes therapy targets in-school behavior. In those cases, teachers have to be part of the process. You'll need to get your child's teacher to agree to help enforce the behavior plan. You'll also need to make sure the plan is simple enough that it won't eat up too much of the teacher's time and attention.

It's important to know that therapy isn't always enough to help with ADHD symptoms. If your child is still struggling, talk to his doctor. Together you can discuss whether to consider ADHD medication in addition to or instead of behavior therapy. You may also want to read about different professionals who help kids with ADHD.

Behavioral Therapy

Chapter 2

Types of Behavioral Therapy

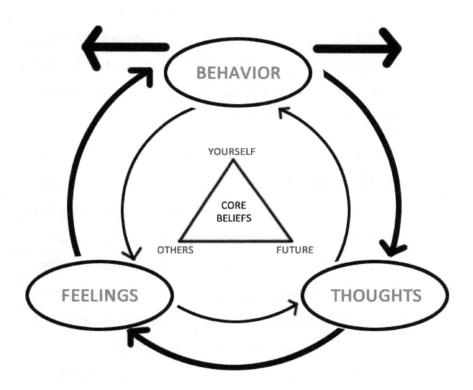

Different types of behavioral therapy techniques exist that behavior therapists utilize to treat mental disorders in both adults and children. Combinations of different treatments are also beneficial, however, any behavioral treatment should be supervised and administered by a behavior therapist or a behavioral therapist.

A. Cognitive Behavioral Therapy

Cognitive-behavioral therapy (CBT) is "a time-sensitive, structured, present-oriented psychotherapy directed toward solving current problems and teaching patients skills to modify dysfunctional behavior."

CBT is a behavior therapy that is based on the cognitive model, which is the way that people perceive a certain event or situation is more closely connected to their reaction than to the situation that is occurring. CBT stresses on the fact that is patients can change the way they think, and they can gain control of their mood. When behavior therapists use CBT for patients over time improvements, and alleviation of symptoms from mental disorders becomes near- constant.

CBT is a very popular behavior therapy technique and is a proven, reliable treatment for mental disorders. CBT is popular because it combines behavioral therapy with cognitive therapy. The main teaching of CBT is how important it is to realize the effect your thoughts and feelings have on your interpretation of certain situations. These factors can also control your mood, which makes CBT an effective choice with people suffering from mental disorders that greatly affect mood.

Behavioral therapists typically have a patient focus on addressing present problems they are going through at the time of therapy. By focusing on how to solve them people develop different reactionary skills when processing similar situations in the future. Developing healthier reactions is key to overcoming symptoms of mental disorders.

Uses for CBT

CBT is an effective way of treating several different mental health conditions.

In addition to depression or anxiety disorders, CBT can also help people with:

- Bipolar disorder
- Borderline personality disorder
- Eating disorders – such as anorexia and bulimia
- Obsessive-compulsive disorder (OCD)

- Panic disorder
- Phobias
- Post-traumatic stress disorder (PTSD)
- Psychosis
- Schizophrenia
- Sleep problems – such as insomnia
- Problems related to alcohol misuse

CBT is also sometimes used to treat people with long-term health conditions, such as:

- Irritable bowel syndrome (IBS)
- Chronic fatigue syndrome (CFS)
- Fibromyalgia

Although CBT cannot cure the physical symptoms of these conditions, it can help people cope better with their symptoms.

What happens during CBT sessions?

If CBT is recommended, you'll usually have a session with a therapist once a week or once every 2 weeks.

The course of treatment usually lasts for between 5 and 20 sessions, with each session lasting 30 to 60 minutes.

Behavioral Therapy

During the sessions, you'll work with your therapist to break down your problems into their separate parts, such as your thoughts, physical feelings, and actions.

You and your therapist will analyze these areas to work out if they're unrealistic or unhelpful and to determine the effect they have on each other and you.

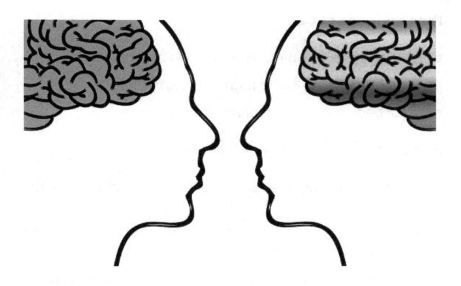

Your therapist will then be able to help you work out how to change unhelpful thoughts and behaviors.

Behavioral Therapy

After working out what you can change, your therapist will ask you to practice these changes in your daily life and you'll discuss how you got on during the next session.

The eventual aim of therapy is to teach you to apply the skills you have learned during treatment to your daily life.

This should help you manage your problems and stop them from having a negative impact on your life, even after your course of treatment finishes.

Pros and cons of CBT

Cognitive-behavioral therapy (CBT) can be as effective as medicine in treating some mental health problems, but it may not be successful or suitable for everyone.

Some of the advantages of CBT include:

- It may be helpful in cases where medication alone has not worked.
- It can be completed in a relatively short period of time compared with other talking therapies.
- The highly structured nature of CBT means it can be provided in different formats, including in groups, self-help books, and apps (you can find mental health apps and tools in the NHS apps library).

- It teaches you useful and practical strategies that can be used in everyday life, even after the treatment has finished.

Some of the disadvantages of CBT to consider include:

- You need to commit yourself to the process to get the most from it – a therapist can help and advise you, but they need your co-operation

- Attending regular CBT sessions and carrying out any extra work between sessions can take up a lot of your time
- It may not be suitable for people with more complex mental health needs or learning difficulties, as it requires structured sessions
- It involves confronting your emotions and anxieties – you may experience initial periods where you're anxious or emotionally uncomfortable

It focuses on the person's capacity to change themselves (their thoughts, feelings, and behaviors) – this does not address any wider problems in systems or families that often have a significant impact on someone's health and wellbeing.

Some critics also argue that because CBT only addresses current problems and focuses on specific issues, it does not address the possible underlying causes of mental health conditions, such as an unhappy childhood.

The Effectiveness of Cognitive Behavioral Therapy

Cognitive Behavioral Therapy (CBT) is an approach that addresses dysfunctional emotions behavior, and cognitive processes based upon a combination of basic behavioral and cognitive principles and techniques. CBT is problem-focused and action-oriented strategy therapists use to help patients address specific problems such as anxiety, depression, and even more complex psychiatric problems.

Cognitive Behavioral Therapy refers to several structured methods of a psychotherapy that center on the thoughts behind a patient's issues. One survey of nearly 2,300 psychologists in the United States found that about 70 percent use CBT in combination with other therapies to treat depression and anxiety. CBT is also a predominant psychotherapy paradigm being taught in psychology graduate degree programs.

How Cognitive Behavioral Therapy Works

Cognitive Behavioral Therapy is based on the idea that human beings are somewhat irrational and make a lot of illogical errors whenever they assess the risks and benefits of various situations and courses of their thoughts and actions. This can lead to out-of-control emotions such as anger and depression. But, CBT is also used to treat a variety more complex issues, such as Post-traumatic Stress Disorder (PTSD), OCD, substance abuse, ADHD, eating disorders, bipolar disorder, among other illnesses.

Cognitive Behavioral Therapists must have a good rapport with their patients for it to be effective such as good communication skills and a good match in personality types. This is because the patient and therapist work together to discuss the issues at hand and the patient's thinking reasonings for his or her thoughts and actions towards those issues. the ultimate goal is to change thinking patterns so the patient can experience fewer chronically negative emotional states.

The National Alliance for Mental Health in favor of CBT because it has excellent scientific data supporting its use in the clinical treatment of mental illness, and it has achieved wide popularity both for therapists and patients alike. A growing number of psychologists, psychiatrists, social workers, and psychiatric nurses have training in CBT.

Research on the effectiveness of CBT is effective for a wide range of disorders. These studies are well- controlled, the data are analyzed sufficiently, and the results speak for themselves. For example, CBT has been found to provide significant advantages in the treatment of bipolar disorder and resulting in fewer days in the hospital, lower rates of suicide, and lower rates of para-suicidal or self-injurious behavior.

Precautions to Take Before Starting Cognitive Behavioral Therapy

Psychiatrists, clinical psychologists, social workers and other mental health professionals complete years of training and education, however, it is possible to practice therapy without such a solid training background. Some things to research before deciding upon a CBT practitioner are educational background and training, along with any professional associations do they belong to, such as the Association for Behavioral and Cognitive Therapies, where most top therapists are members.

Before seeing a making your first appointment, check his or her background, education, certification, and licensing. A psychotherapist is often used as a general term. Make sure that the therapist you choose meets state certification and licensing requirements for his or her particular discipline. The key is to find a skilled therapist who can match the type and therapy with your needs. In most cases, CBT is most effective when it is combined with other treatments, such as taking medications. So, in addition to your therapist, you might also need a psychiatrist for prescribing medications.

Another thing to consider is cost. If you have health insurance, find out what coverage it offers for the therapy sessions. Some health plans cover only a certain number of therapy sessions a year. Some may not be covered at all. So, be sure to talk to the therapist about fees and payment options before your first visit.

Before your first appointment, think about what problems you are having that need treatment. While you can also sort some of this out with your therapist, having a good sense of your problems in advance can help as a starting point. Again, check for their qualifications and experience, specifically with your issues. Some therapists may not meet the qualifications you need. If you do not find the right one the first time around, do not give up. Do your homework, and you will be able to find a good Cognitive Behavioral Therapist.

The History of Cognitive Behavioral Therapy

Cognitive-behavioral therapy is an approach used by psychotherapists to influence a patient's behaviors and emotions. The key to the approach is in its procedure which must be systematic. It has been used successfully to treat a variety of disorders including eating disorders, substance abuse, anxiety and personality disorders. It can be used in individual or group therapy sessions and the approach can also be geared towards self-help therapy.

Cognitive-behavioral therapy is a combination of traditional behavioral therapy and cognitive therapy. They are combined into a treatment that is focused on symptom removal. The effectiveness of the treatment can clearly be judged based on its results. The more it is used, the more it has become recommended. It is now used as the number one treatment technique for post-traumatic stress disorder, obsessive-compulsive disorder, depression, and bulimia.

Cognitive-behavioral therapy first began to be used between 1960 and 1970. It was a gradual process of merging behavioral therapy techniques and cognitive therapy techniques. Behavioral therapy had been around since the

1920s, but cognitive therapy was not introduced until the 1960s. Almost immediately the benefits of combining it with behavioral therapy techniques were realized. Ivan Pavlov, with his dogs who salivated at the ringing of the dinner bell, was among the most famous of the behavioral research pioneers. Other leaders in the field included John Watson and Clark Hull.

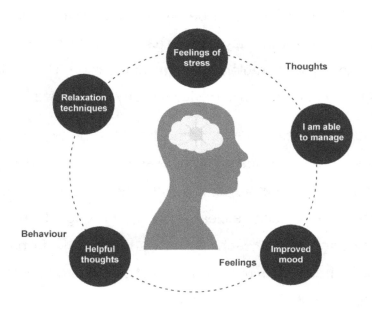

Instead of focusing on analyzing the problem like Freud and the psychoanalysts, cognitive behavioral therapy focused on eliminating the symptoms. The idea is that if you eliminate the symptoms, you have eliminated the problem. This more direct approach was seen as more effective at getting to the problem at hand and helping patients to make progress more quickly.

As a more radical aggressive treatment, behavioral techniques dealt better with more radical problems. The more obvious and clear cut the symptoms were, the easier it was to target them and devise treatments to eliminate them. Behavioral therapy was not as successful initially with more ambiguous problems such as depression. This realm was better served with cognitive therapy techniques.

In many academic settings, the two therapy techniques were used side by side to compare and contrast the results. It was not long before the advantages of combining the two techniques became clear as a way of taking advantage of the strengths of each. David Barlow's work on panic disorder treatments provided the first concrete example of the success of the combined strategies.

Cognitive-behavioral therapy is difficult to define in a succinct definition because it covers such a broad range of topics and techniques. It is really an umbrella definition for individual treatments that are specifically tailored to the problems of a specific patient. So the problem dictates the specifics of the treatment, but there are some common themes and techniques. These include having the patient keep a diary of important events and record the feelings and behaviors they had in association with each event. This tool is then used as a basis to analyze and test the patient's ability to evaluate the situation and develop an appropriate emotional response. Negative emotions and behaviors are identified as well as the evaluations and beliefs that lead to them. An effort is then made to counter these beliefs and evaluations to show that the resulting behaviors are wrong. Negative behaviors are eliminated and the patient is taught a better way to view and react to the situation.

Part of the therapy also includes teaching the patient ways to distract themselves or change their focus from something that is upsetting or a situation that is generating negative behavior. They learn to focus on something else instead of the negative stimulus, thus eliminating the negative behavior that it would lead to. The problem is essentially nipped in the bud. For serious psychological disorders like bipolar disorder or schizophrenia, mood-stabilizing medications are often prescribed to use in conjunction with these techniques. The medications give the patient enough of a calming effect to give them the opportunity to examine the situation and make a healthy choice whereas before they could not even pause for rational thought.

Cognitive-behavioral therapy has been proven effective for a variety of problems, but it is still a process, not a miracle cure. It takes time to teach patients to understand situations and identify the triggers of their negative behaviors. Once this step is mastered, it still takes a lot of effort to overcome their first instincts and instead stop and make the right choices. First, they learn what they should do, and then they must practice until they can do it.

Principles of Cognitive Behavioral Therapy

Cognitive-behavioral therapy, or CBT, is a psychotherapy technique that attempts to teach patients to correct emotional and behavioral responses to troubling situations. The treatment focuses on identifying the situations that lead to negative emotions and behaviors and then examining the thought process and beliefs of the patient that leads them to make the wrong behavioral choices. Once patients are aware that they are making the wrong choice and understand why they can be retrained to make the right choices with the result being the elimination of the negative behavior. This is always the goal of CBT: to eliminate the negative behavior.

The treatment is effective when it is done as a systematic process and it takes time. Patients need to encounter problem situations numerous times to have the opportunity to retrain their thinking and thereby change their behaviors. Cognitive-behavioral therapy has been successful in the treatment of eating disorders, anxiety, insomnia, obsessive-compulsive disorder, and post-traumatic stress disorder.

Cognitive-behavioral therapy had its beginnings in the 1960s when advances in behavioral therapy, which had been around since the 1920s, was combined with the new field of cognitive therapy. Both techniques had their strengths and weaknesses but combining the two seemed to be the best of both worlds. As long as the patient had significant cognitive functions to understand the underlying assumptions that were responsible for their negative behaviors, then they could be retrained to assess the situation more correctly and generate a different emotion or behavior as a response in place of the negative one.

Each individual creates their unique view of any given situation. This view is based in part on our past experiences as other environmental factors. For some people, this view is distorted and that leads them to an irrational response to the situation. Given their distorted view, this response may seem to be perfectly acceptable. Therefore the first step in cognitive behavioral therapy is to teach people to view the trouble situations clearly so that they can then learn the correct appropriate reaction.

This approach which directly engages the patient's behaviors is in stark contrast to the psychoanalysts approach like that pioneered by Freud. Freud's techniques look backward, searching out the root of the problem, while cognitive-behavioral therapy looks forward to the result and starts there. The theory being that if you eliminate the symptoms, then you have effectively cured the disorder. CBT requires repetition to teach patients the appropriate responses to stimuli and to help them understand how to make that right choice so they can apply those new decision-making skills to real-life situations.

In this way, cognitive behavioral therapy owes a debt to early behavioral researchers like Ivan Pavlov who among his many experiments showed that dogs could be trained to salivate at the sound of a bell if the sound was repeatedly associated with their mealtime. In the same way, positive behaviors are trained into patients until that hopefully becomes their natural response instead of the negative behavior that brought them to therapy in the first place.

For the therapist, the key to solving a patient's behavioral problems lies in uncovering the underlying assumptions that the patient holds that act as a trigger for the behavior. Once the therapist has identified these flawed assumptions, they can help the patient change them. Once the patient understands that the assumptions they held were wrong, they can be replaced with correct ones. Once this transformation occurs, the patients' reactions to situations will also change and the negative, inappropriate behavior will be eliminated.

Given the types of assumptions or even core beliefs that the therapist is asking the patient to question and ultimately change, the situation can naturally be quite volatile. For this reason, these techniques take time. A therapist does not want to shake a patient's belief to the core without giving them something else to build upon so the therapist must move slowly in steps. Validity testing is a common first step, where the patient is asked to explain or defend his or her beliefs or assumptions. If they are faulty, then eventually the patient will see the flaws in the logic. The therapist cannot simply tell the patient this however, the patient has to learn it on their own so they understand it as well as accept it.

The results of cognitive behavioral therapy show that the lengthy process is worth the effort because, in the end, it is effective. That is why cognitive behavioral therapy is the number one treatment for a wide variety of disorders from bulimia to panic disorder.

Cognitive-Behavioral Therapy - The Basics

Cognitive-Behavioral Therapy is a form of psychotherapy that emphasizes the important role of thinking in how we feel and what we do.

Cognitive-behavioral therapy does not exist as a distinct therapeutic technique. The term "cognitive- behavioral therapy (CBT)" is a very general term for a classification of therapies with similarities. There are several approaches to cognitive-behavioral therapy, including Rational Emotive Behavior Therapy, Rational Behavior Therapy, Rational Living Therapy, Cognitive Therapy, and Dialectic Behavior Therapy.

However, most cognitive-behavioral therapies have the following characteristics:

1. CBT is based on the Cognitive Model of Emotional Response

    Cognitive-behavioral therapy is based on the idea that our thoughts cause our feelings and behaviors, not external things, like people, situations, and events. The benefit of this fact is that we can change the way we think to feel/act better even if the situation does not change.

2. CBT is Briefer and Time-Limited

    Cognitive-behavioral therapy is considered among the most rapid in terms of results obtained. The average number of sessions clients receive (across all types of problems and approaches to CBT) is only 16. Other forms of therapy, like psychoanalysis, can take years. What enables CBT to be briefer is its highly instructive nature and the fact that it makes use of homework assignments. CBT is time-limited in that we help clients understand at the very beginning of the therapy process that there will be a point when the formal therapy will end. The ending of formal therapy is a decision made by the therapist and client. Therefore, CBT is not an open-ended, never-ending process.

3. A sound therapeutic relationship is necessary for effective therapy, but not the focus. Some forms of therapy assume that the main reason people get better in therapy is because of the positive relationship between the therapist and client. Cognitive-behavioral therapists believe it is important to have a good, trusting relationship, but that is not enough. CBT therapists believe that the clients change because they learn how to think differently and they act on that learning. Therefore, CBT therapists focus on teaching rational self-counseling skills.

4. CBT is a collaborative effort between the therapist and the client

Cognitive-behavioral therapists seek to learn what their clients want out of life (their goals) and then help their clients achieve those goals. The therapist's role is to listen, teach, and encourage, while the client's roles are to express concerns, learn, and implement that learning.

5. CBT is based on Stoic philosophy

Not all approaches to CBT emphasize stoicism. Rational Emotive Behavior Therapy, Rational Behavior Therapy, and Rational Living Therapy emphasize stoicism. Beck's Cognitive Therapy is not based on stoicism. Cognitive-behavioral therapy does not tell people how they should feel. However, most people seeking therapy do not want to feel the way they have been feeling. The approaches that emphasize stoicism teaches the benefits of feeling, at worst, calm when confronted with undesirable situations. They also emphasize the fact that we have our undesirable situations whether we are upset about them or not. If we are upset about our problems, we have two problems -- the problem, and our upset about it. Most people want to have the fewest number of problems possible. So when we learn how to more calmly accept a personal problem, not only do we feel better, but we usually put ourselves in a better position to make use of our intelligence, knowledge, energy, and resources to resolve the problem.

6. CBT uses the Socratic Method

Cognitive-behavioral therapists want to gain a very good understanding of their clients' concerns. That's why they often ask questions. They also encourage their clients to ask questions of themselves, like, "How do I really know that those people are laughing at me?" "Could they be laughing about something else?"

7. CBT is structured and directive

Cognitive-behavioral therapists have a specific agenda for each session. Specific techniques/concepts are taught during each session. CBT focuses on the client's goals. We do not tell our clients what their goals "should" be, or what they "should" tolerate. We are directive in the sense that we show our clients how to think and behave in ways to obtain what they want. Therefore, CBT therapists do not tell their clients what to do -- rather, they teach their clients how to do.

8. CBT is based on an educational model

> CBT is based on the scientifically supported assumption that most emotional and behavioral reactions are learned. Therefore, the goal of therapy is to help clients unlearn their unwanted reactions and to learn a new way of reacting. Therefore, CBT has nothing to do with "just talking". People can "just talk" with anyone. The educational emphasis of CBT has an additional benefit -- it leads to long term results. When people understand how and why they are doing well, they know what to do to continue doing well.

9. CBT theory and techniques rely on the Inductive Method

> A central aspect of Rational thinking is that it is based on fact. Often, we upset ourselves about things when, in fact, the situation isn't like we think it is. If we knew that, we would not waste our time upsetting ourselves. Therefore, the inductive method encourages us to look at our thoughts as being

hypotheses or guesses that can be questioned and tested. If we find that our hypotheses are incorrect (because we have new information), then we can change our thinking to be in line with how the situation really is.

10. Homework is a central feature of CBT

If when you attempted to learn your multiplication tables you spent only one hour per week studying them, you might still be wondering what 5 X 5 equals. You very likely spent a great deal of time at home studying your multiplication tables, maybe with flashcards. The same is the case with psychotherapy. Goal achievement (if obtained) could take a very long time if all a person were only to think about the techniques and topics taught was for one hour per week. That's why CBT therapists assign reading assignments and encourage their clients to practice the techniques learned.

What Constitutes Cognitive Behavioral Therapy?

Cognitive-behavioral therapy is a psychotherapeutic approach that aims to teach a person new skills on how to solve problems concerning dysfunctional emotions, behaviors, and cognitions through a goal-oriented, systematic approach. This title is used in many ways to differentiate behavioral therapy, cognitive therapy, and therapy that is based on both behavioral and cognitive therapies. There is empirical evidence that shows that cognitive-behavioral therapy is quite effective in treating several conditions, including personality, anxiety, mood, eating, substance abuse, and psychotic disorders. Treatment is often manualized, as specific psychological orders are treated with specific technique-driven brief, direct, and time-limited treatments.

Cognitive-behavioral therapy can be used both with individuals and in groups. The techniques are often adapted for self-help sessions as well. It is up to the individual clinician or researcher on whether he/she is more cognitive oriented, more behavioral oriented, or a combination of both, as all three methods are used today. Cognitive-behavioral therapy was born out of a combination of behavioral therapy and cognitive therapy. These two therapies have many differences, but found common ground on focusing on the "here and now" and on alleviating symptoms.

Evaluating cognitive behavioral therapy has led to many believing that it is more effective over psychodynamic treatments and other methods. The United Kingdom advocates the use of cognitive- behavioral therapy over other methods for many mental health difficulties, including post-traumatic stress disorder, obsessive-compulsive disorder, bulimia nervosa, clinical depression, and the neurological condition chronic fatigue syndrome/myalgic encephalomyelitis. The precursors of cognitive-behavioral therapy base their roots in various ancient philosophical traditions, especially Stoicism. The modern roots of CBT can be traced to the development of behavioral therapy in the 1920s, the development of cognitive therapy in the 1960s, and the subsequent merging of the two

therapies. The first behavioral therapeutic approaches were published in 1924 by Mary Cover Jones, whose work dealt with the unlearning of fears in children.

The early behavioral approaches worked well with many of the neurotic disorders, but not so much with depression. Behavioral therapy was also losing in popularity due to the "cognitive revolution." This eventually led to cognitive therapy being founded by Aaron T. Beck in the 1960s. The first form of cognitive-behavioral therapy was developed by Arnold A. Lazarus during the period of the late 1950s through the 1970s. During the 1980s and 1990s, cognitive and behavioral therapies were combined by work done by David M. Clark in the United Kingdom and David H. Barlow in the United States. Cognitive-behavioral therapy includes the following systems: cognitive therapy, rational emotive behavior therapy, and multimodal therapy. One of the greatest challenges is defining exactly what cognitive-behavioral therapy is. The particular therapeutic techniques vary within the different approaches of CBT depending upon what kind of problem issues are being dealt with, but the techniques usually center around the following:

- Keeping a diary of significant events and associated feelings, thoughts, and behaviors.
- Questioning and testing cognitions, evaluations, assumptions, and beliefs that might be unrealistic and unhelpful.
- Gradually facing activities that may have been avoided.
- Trying out new ways of behaving and reacting.

Also, distraction techniques, mindfulness, and relaxation are commonly used in cognitive behavioral therapy. Mood-stabilizing medications are also often combined with therapies to treat conditions like bipolar disorder. The NICE guidelines within the British NHS recognize cognitive behavioral therapy's application in treating schizophrenia in combination with medication and therapy. Cognitive-behavioral therapy usually takes time for patients to effectively implement it into their lives. It usually takes concentrated effort for them to replace a dysfunctional cognitive-affective- behavioral process or habit with a more reasonable and adaptive one, even when they recognize when and where their mental processes go awry. Cognitive-behavioral therapy is applied to many different situations, including the following conditions:

Anxiety disorders (obsessive-compulsive disorder, social phobia or social anxiety, generalized
anxiety disorder)

- Mood disorders (clinical depression, major depressive disorder, psychiatric symptoms)
- Insomnia (including being more effective than the drug Zopiclone)
- Severe mental disorders (schizophrenia, bipolar disorder, severe depression)
- Children and adolescents (major depressive disorder, anxiety disorders, trauma, and

posttraumatic stress disorder symptoms)
- Stuttering (to help them overcome anxiety, avoidance behaviors, and negative thoughts about themselves)

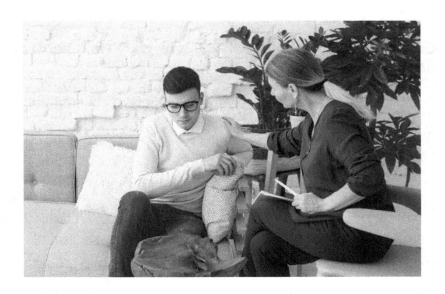

Cognitive-behavioral therapy involves teaching a person new skills to overcome dysfunctional emotions, behaviors, and cognitions through a goal-oriented, systematic approach. There is empirical evidence showing that cognitive-behavioral therapy is effective in treating many conditions, including obsessive-compulsive disorder, generalized anxiety disorder, major depressive disorder, schizophrenia, anxiety, and negative thoughts about oneself). With the vast amount of success shown by the use of this therapy, it is one of the most important tools that researchers and therapists have to treat mental disorders today.

Cognitive Behavioral Therapy and the Treatment of Addiction

Addiction can take many forms: alcoholism, substance abuse, gambling addiction, etc. The list goes on. The question that needs to be answered is how can these addictions be eliminated? Nowadays, with the technology boom, online meetings for treating addiction is available as well as online counseling and other forms of treatment. One of the oldest addiction treatments is the twelve-step program developed by the founders of Alcoholics Anonymous. In these modern times, however, other treatment programs are being practiced such as the so-called Cognitive Behavioral Therapy that a user undergoes if he/she wants to be sober.

Cognitive Behavioral Therapy (CBT) is a member of a branch of psychotherapy that gives importance to how a person thinks. It follows that what is on the person's mind will greatly affect the actions and the feelings of the individual. Several programs under cognitive behavioral therapy include Rational Living Therapy, Rational Emotive Behavior Therapy, Cognitive Therapy, Rational Behavior Therapy, and Dialectic Behavior Therapy.

CBT is now being applied in treating alcoholism and substance abuse. It works in the following ways:

- It is based on the asking questions (Socrates' method)
- An emotional response is given importance in Cognitive Behavioral Therapy, wherein the belief that changing the way a user thinks will make that person feel better as well as act better (e.g. if the user thinks of staying clean for a year, then that will be done successfully).

Behavioral Therapy

- In CBT, the client and the therapist should interact harmoniously and should trust each other for the treatment to be successful
- In CBT, users feel that they are in control because they are made to analyze their actions and they would be the ones to make decisions on the steps they would take. If they feel that a mistake was made, it's up to them to correct it.
- The most commonly used CBT program that battles addiction is Rational Emotive Behavioral Therapy (REBT). It focuses on providing solutions to disturbances and problems that are behavioral as well as emotional in nature that aims to lead to a satisfied and happy individual.
- REBT applies the A-B-C-model of psychological disturbance and change. This model believes that the things that people believe in are the main reasons why people are disturbed, and should not be blamed on the adversities that are experienced by the alcoholics or drug addicts. In this model, the users are taught to examine the things they believe in and do the best they can to turn those beliefs into something that would produce positive results.

- Take note that REBT is considered to be a brief therapy that is there to solve specific problems. More complex problems require longer therapy. The REBT therapist aids the user in improving oneself through hard work that would also help the person overcome trials and obstacles. At the end of the therapy, the user is expected to feel self-acceptance as well as the acceptance of life's realities.
- It is said that severe alcoholism and addiction problems can be treated with Cognitive Behavioral Therapy. Its structured teaching method aims to improve on the way the patients deal with life. It is also an effective way to improve the user's way of thinking in terms of drinking.

How Can Cognitive-Behavioral Therapy Help OCD Sufferers?

The suffering of many people from Obsessive-Compulsive Disorder (OCD) has led to numerous studies and researches, most of which aim to find means to treat, if not cure, OCD. One of the most popular methods of treatment practiced today is the use of Cognitive-Behavioral Therapy (CBT). This therapy is a form of psychotherapy which capitalizes on the value of thinking in addressing how an individual feels and does.

CBT is the general term for any therapeutic technique which uses the mind -- common examples are the Rational Emotive Therapy, Rational Living Therapy, Dielectric Behavior Therapy, Cognitive Therapy, and Rational Behavior Therapy. Though all these types of therapies are unique form each other in terms of specific performance, some characteristics of these therapies are uniform to all.

One characteristic common to all is the idea that all cognitive-behavioral therapies are based on the cognitive model of emotional response. This means that the therapy is centered on the principle that all our feelings and behaviors are internally modeled; it further implies that these are caused by our thoughts and not of any pressure or influence from our environment. The conclusion to this is that despite the fact that situations may not change, the way we think about the situation can.

Another characteristic is the brevity of the therapies. All cognitive-behavioral therapies would take a maximum of 16 sessions only to complete. This is made possible by making the patient thoroughly understand the nature of his or her condition and that the therapy will end at a specific time agreed upon by the therapist and the patient. Such mental conditioning makes the patient more cooperative to the goal of the therapy and all experts agree that this is in fact what OCD treatments need most -- cooperation from patients.

All CBTs also revolve around the principle that for the therapy to be effective and efficient is to make the patient believe that he or she can think differently through rational self-counseling skills. It is a collaborative effort between the CBT therapist and the OCD sufferer. The therapist's role involves the expression of concern towards the condition of the sufferer, listening to his or her woes, teaching him or her how to get through the entire process and encouraging him or her that he or she has every capacity to succeed in the therapy.

To make the recovering process more efficient, CBT also includes giving assignments and readings to the sufferer from which he or she can learn for himself or herself how to do self-control and how to privately practice the neutralizing activities he is encouraged to do when his or her obsessions compel him or her to do OCD rituals. This way, CBT is by far the fastest-growing OCD treatment in terms of popularity and preference by many OCD sufferers.

Cognitive Behavioral Therapy for Treating Autism

Several behavioral therapies have been tried from time to time for treating children with autism. Pivotal response training and applied behavior analysis are two of the most commons. But adults, older children, and teens are likely to benefit more from cognitive behavioral therapy, another major intervention to treat autism.

There have been many attempts to adapt cognitive-behavioral therapy for teens and older children having autism. The target has usually been on those who suffer from anxiety as well because this is a common trait in autism. The challenge has been to find out whether autistic children have skills that are required for cognitive behavioral therapy to be a success. The response, fortunately, is in the

affirmative. A 2012 study, evaluated the cognitive skills of older children with autism and compared them with those of non-autistic children. Almost every child in the former group had cognitive behavioral skills and they could distinguish feelings, behaviors, and thoughts. They only found difficult to recognize emotions.

Behavioral Therapy

Traditional cognitive behavioral therapy calls for strong language and abstract thinking capabilities, and this is often a challenge for those having autism. Researchers have realized this and have modified the therapy to suit autistic people, like making it more visually appealing and concrete, and repetitive. For instance, merely asking the children to orally rank their anxiety on a scale of one to 10, a therapist may have a thermometer that shows the anxiety level from low to high, and ask the participants indicate the prop for illustrating this. Another strategy in cognitive behavioral therapy for autism involves focusing on a child's talent and special interests that help to keep the children motivated and engaged and build frequent sensory activities and movement breaks for those who may have attention deficit problems with under or over-reactivity.

The researchers noted that cognitive behavior therapy must address social skills among those with autism because core social deficits among young persons with autism contribute to anxiety which then goes on to intensify the teen's social problems.

The therapy can be delivered in several ways, like family, individual, groups, and even both families and groups.

Group therapies have the advantage that an individual with autism can see similar other people struggling with the same difficulties and trying to overcome them together. Social support and friendship gained through the process could be healing in themselves.

A family behavioral therapy for autism often involves parents who educate themselves about their children's challenges. It also involves teaching them to encourage using cognitive behavioral therapy techniques when a real-life situation confronts the child. This will make them feel confident and hopeful for contributing a positive change in a child's life.

Researchers have found that the issue of protecting children from a potentially negative experience, is often a tough call for most parents. Autistic children usually have a history of behavioral and emotional challenges and painful real failures in the world. Their parents are often reluctant to expose the child to further failures, and inadvertently limit the exposure to experiences necessary to become less anxious and more independent.

Cognitive Behavioral Therapy for Anxiety - Does It Work?

Behavioral Therapy

Will cognitive behavioral therapy for anxiety be effective? Understanding the methodology behind this type of therapy is an important first step to answering this question. CBT is typically engaged in for a specific period and with a specific goal in mind, unlike talk therapy or psychoanalysis, which could continue for years. The goal is to modify thoughts that underlie unwanted behaviors.

Cognitive Behavioral Therapy is founded on the premise that behaviors are responses to our thoughts, rather than responses to external events. Because thoughts are learned, we can isolate and unlearn our negative thoughts. After we are able to establish a positive pattern of thinking, our negative reactions will stop. Under the care of a professional therapist, cognitive behavioral therapy breaks down a big problem into smaller, more manageable problems. This allows the patient and therapist to work together to resolve these smaller issues. For example:

Jim is a hypochondriac. He deals with imaginary aches and pains daily. He visits his doctor frequently with new symptoms for which the doctor can find no cause; nevertheless, Jim continues to be certain that he has a life-threatening problem. Jim puts a lot of time in on the internet, searching websites for more information about various symptoms and illnesses.

Jim and his CBT therapist would go through a process of isolating and articulating his negative thoughts, and then putting positive thoughts in their place. Jim and his therapist might come up with this solution:

"The aches and pains are all in my mind. I know my body is strong and healthy because it has been fully checked out by my doctor. Because I am confident in my good health, I am looking forward to getting back to active living. I will let my pains go because they are not in my body, but rather in my mind. Instead of simply going home and going to bed, I intend to revel in my newfound strength and vitality by going on an energetic walk."

This illustrates the process of replacing negative with positive thoughts in order to modify behaviors, even though it is an extremely optimistic example. It is easy to see that cognitive behavioral therapy for anxiety does have potential to help sufferers. Working with a trained therapist is critical to the success of a CBT approach. People who suffer from anxiety often hold onto their beliefs with a lot of conviction. Trying new and more healthy ways of thinking is what the trained professional will be coaxing the patient to do. This type of therapy would be extremely challenging were it not for that professional guidance.

So is there a self-help way to do cognitive behavioral therapy for anxiety? Strictly speaking, no. But framing solutions much like CBT is an approach that is common with several self-help options. Such an approach includes:

- Identify negative thinking
- Acknowledge that perceived threats are in your mind -- not real.
- Look for another approach to thinking that points to healthier behaviors.

As you are considering your self-help options, it will be useful to understand the components of cognitive-behavioral therapy. Cognitive-behavioral therapy for anxiety can be expensive, so for this and many other reasons, a sufferer may want to select a self-help option. Look for options that focus on the current problem (not options that delve into a person's past) and for options that encourage the sufferer to move slowly and thoughtfully toward healthier mental patterns. Neither CBT nor similar solutions are fast fixes. Even though cognitive behavioral therapy for anxiety takes time and effort, it is not as lengthy a process as some other forms of therapy. With dedication and perseverance, cognitive behavioral therapy for anxiety can and does work for many people.

Can Cognitive Behavioral Therapy Be Useful For Anger Management?

As we choose to make our lives more updated and in-tune with the times, we end up piling on endless chores to fit in our limited 24-hour schedule. Attempting to accomplish everything within a limited period is what we are left doing, accommodating almost any and everything into a single day. We all want to earn, learn and have fun 'altogether' often not to realize the aftermaths. Stress, rage, and anger all stem from our no-idle time routines. And, this is happening all over the world. With each passing day, we have an increasing number of violent incidents being reported. The number of angry kids, angry parents, angry spouses, angry bosses and angry workers is increasing unstoppably. And, 'anger' is passed down the generations. So, where this will stop is virtually hard to fathom.

While a variety of correctional techniques are being employed to address this situation and curb the growing number of angry individuals, Cognitive Behavioral Therapy or CBT promises best results especially when it comes to curing behavioral problems including anger. Anger is a behavioral problem but a natural human expression too. We get angry when something that happens does not match our standards of perfection or as a result of continuing negative emotions of low self-esteem, jealousy, rejection, abuse or exposure to life-threatening conditions. When you lose control over an angry moment, accidents happen. It is then we should opt for treatment. One may never feel the need

to go in for treatment either thinking he'll grow out of that or that will make him feel rather low. But, whatever the cause be, treatment must never be denied or postponed.

Cognitive Behavioral Therapy targets a direct alteration in the thinking process of a patient. Anger results from negative emotions. Cognitive Behavioral Therapy helps controls the generation of negative emotions and events that cause such emotions such that anger may never find a place in a person's life ever again.

Cognitive Behavioral Therapy adopts a variety of approaches and systems to help correct the behavioral problems of an individual. Some of the most employed techniques being Acceptance and Commitment Therapy,

Behavioral Therapy

Applied Behavioral Analysis, Exposure and response prevention, Multimodal Therapy, Problem-Solving Therapy, Rational Emotive Behavior Therapy and more that basically focus on relaxation and assertiveness. Cognitive Behavioral Therapy involves:

- Identifying behavioral problems
- Identifying the triggers to negative feelings resulting in behavioral problems
- Devising ways to curb negative feelings
- Designing alternate reactions and behavioral patterns
- Practicing and
- Finally treating the cause of negative emotions by altering the emotional schema of a person to avoid a relapse.

Anger can be managed and managed better with Cognitive Behavioral Therapy. It is only when you entrust your therapist and therapy will you be able to manage this extremely difficult situation easily. However, if you still feel uncomfortable visiting a doctor for therapy, you may consider Computerized CBT in which you will interact with a computer software installed on a computer or through voice - activated phone service, instead of an individual. In most cases, all we need is expressing our innermost feelings to someone, then let it be a therapist or a software. All that matters is the cure.

Using Cognitive Behavior Therapy (CBT) for Panic Attacks

If you want to seek treatment that involves talking and counseling, Cognitive Behavioral Therapy (CBT) has been found to be a successful route for around half of people who suffer from panic attacks or agoraphobia. Cognitive Behavioral Therapy aims to change your thoughts and behavior and is statistically proven to have a high success rate when treating anxiety, panic attacks, and phobias.

Cognitive Behavioral Therapy works because it attempts to both help you process why you may be having the thoughts you have leading up to a panic attack and then help you change your behaviors to help you manage them with your state feeling one build up. CBT is made of two elements, cognitive therapy, and behavior therapy.

Cognitive therapy is based on the idea that the way we think triggers panic attacks. Any harmful or unbeneficial thinking patterns are worked through and identified along with false beliefs or thoughts you may have. This will teaches the sufferer to notice their thought patterns, and understand how they are misinterpreting events and causing automatic negative thoughts to spiral out of control resulting in anxiety and panic building up.

Behavior Therapy targets the way you react to things which trigger anxiety, or feelings you associate with the onset of anxiety. The therapist will help you to walk through those scenarios that trigger an attack and help you feel more confident and in control, reducing the prevalences of a panic attack in these situations. This may include the use of mantras or breathing techniques.

CBT is widely used to cure an anxiety disorder, and this is a method to re-program your mind reaction to the trigger of anxiety attacks. However, it won't be solved in one or two sessions especially if the panic disorder is a well-established part of your everyday life.

A. Behavioral Activation Therapy

Behavioral activation therapy is essentially a behavior treatment for depression that aims to target reactions or behaviors tha might maintain or worsen the depression. Behavioral activation therapy model proposes that life events (including loss of life or significant trauma, genetic predispositions to mental disorders like depression or anxiety, and even the hassles in life) lead to people experiencing low amounts of positive reinforcement from their environment. Through a process of negative reinforcement detrimental behaviors used to cope with short-term issues, but in turn are negative in the long-term, increase.

The main issue with the negative reactions to situations is that they tend to increase the symptoms of mental disorders. For example, shutting oneself out and away from everyone and anything might seem like a great idea at the moment when feelings of depression take hold, but in the long run that behavior can only make depression symptoms more severe.

BA proposes an "outside-in" approach utilizing the scheduling of behavior therapy activities aimed to allow patients to begin to increase their chance of having a better opportunity to receive positive reinforcement.

Behavioral analytic theory "recognizes that the outcome or function of a behavior is more important than the form of the behavior". Further, BA targets "avoidance" reactions and behaviors. Avoiding behaviors have to be addressed with proper BA behavioral therapy techniques aimed to alleviate systems of mental disorders in patients.

Behavioral Therapy for Autism

Behavioral therapy for autism has a high chance of success. In this type of treatment, appropriate behavior is rewarded while inappropriate behavior is ignored. The success rate increases if the therapy is started when your child is still young; that is usually before he turns 3-years-old.

You would probably have discovered that your autistic child will challenge your parenting skills with their extremes of behavior. Extremes of behavior would include such things as temper tantrums, self- injurious behavior, aggression, and agitation. Essentially, he is dictating to you what he wants and his preferences. If he does not get what he wants, you are made to suffer the consequences. Rather than giving in, you should learn how to teach your child a more appropriate way in which to get what he wants.

This is where a consistent program of behavioral modification will work very well. It will not only help you to cope with your child's behaviors but it will also teach your child more socially appropriate behaviors. Such a program

Behavioral Therapy

must consist of 4 components: a structured daily routine; behavioral control; communication; and applied behavioral analysis.

You should instill a structured daily routine as your autistic child can then know what to expect. Autistic children do not usually cope well with inconsistency or change. Therefore, sticking to a daily routine is important as much as possible.

The next thing that a parent must learn is how to control tantrums and other such behavioral issues. In doing so there are 3 factors to bear in mind:

1. Those behaviors that are dangerous to the child or those around him must be dealt with first. These behaviors need to immediately be stopped with firm words and actions. Try not to show your child any anger while doing this though.

2. Autistic children need to be taught how to sit. The best way in which to do this is to reward appropriate sitting behavior while either ignoring or giving a negative consequence for inappropriate sitting behavior.

Behavioral Therapy

3. Autistic children tend to have bizarre, stereotypical, repetitive behaviors. The most obvious of these are finger flapping and rocking. These can be very distracting and thus a firm "stop" command is suggested for use. Next direct your child to another activity that will not allow him to continue these behaviors.

It is important that you talk to your child regularly. Whenever you are talking to an autistic child you need to be both simple and direct. You need to use short, clear sentences without going into explanations or using too many words. So, instead of telling your child, "Come here so that I can fix your pants and tuck in your shirt because you need to look nice" simply tell him, "Come here now." This is an easy command to process as you want to avoid confusing him.

Applied behavioral analysis (ABA) is a form of behavioral therapy that is popular. This involves breaking down tasks into individual components. Then, whenever a child successfully completes each step of the task he should be rewarded. It is believed that this form of therapy has a 47% success rate. It is important to note that ABA is not the only behavioral approach to treating autism nor is it a cure for autism. But it is a therapy that should be explored as one of your many options in helping your autistic child.

Behavioral Therapy to Cure Panic Disorder

Proper medical assistance can cure panic disorder at 100%. The treatment of panic disorder consists of two aspects, namely medication and therapy. In many cases, medical professionals specialized in the treatment of panic disorder prefer to bypass medication and focus mainly on therapy as the cure to the said mental illness. They would usually have recourse to two specific therapeutic methods, that is cognitive and behavioral therapy. Cognitive therapy focuses on getting the patient acquainted with every aspect of the illness - including symptoms, triggers, and consequences. Behavioral therapy, on the other hand, centers on correcting particular aspects of the patient's behavior that may be contributing to worsening her or his condition.

Patients suffering from panic disorder, in fact, fear possible attacks more than specific events or objects that are likely to trigger a panic attack. For example, a person with panic disorder may fear air travel not because he/she thinks that the plane will crash but due to the mere thought that he/she may suffer from a panic attack in the place. Behavioral therapy is used to deal with this kind of situational avoidance manifest in patients with panic disorder. An important aspect of the behavioral therapy which people with the panic disorder condition need to go through is what clinicians have termed as 'interoceptive exposure'. This therapy works around the physical sensations that the patient experiences during a panic attack to acquaint the patient with the same and help her or him build up defense mechanisms. Thus the patient feels empowered against eventual attacks and more confident to confront them, which evidently decreases the fear of attacks. The patients also gain better control over their conditions as they realize that every manifestation of a symptom does not always lead to a full-blown panic attack.

This technique of behavioral therapy is similar to a technique known as 'systematic desensitization', and which forms part of therapies against phobias. One effective treatment for phobias is what is clinically termed as 'in vivo exposure'. This therapy consists of breaking down a fearful situation into small manageable steps to gain better mastery over every level of the situation. The same technique is used to help people with panic disorder gain better control

over every phase that they undergo during a panic attack. Relaxation techniques - such as breathing techniques and positive visualization
- are taught to them, which they should then practice during an attack. In fact, during an attack people who suffer from the condition of panic disorder usually experience accelerated breathing rates and heartbeats. Hence, learning to slow down their breathing does help a lot. After ten to twenty sessions of behavioral therapy, improvements can be noticed in the way patients live through an attack. These sessions are usually dispensed every week. Although there are support groups that welcome patients of panic disorder to practice some simple behavioral exercises and techniques during group sessions, the most appropriate techniques can only be learned from a qualified medical practitioner.

B. Aversion Therapy

Other mental issues that proper behavior therapy can address are those that suffer from drug or substance abuse and alcoholism. Aversion therapy can be administered by a behavior therapist, and it aims to teach patients to associate a stimulus that is desirable, yet destructive with another extremely unpleasant stimulus.

The goal of aversion therapy is to teach a patient to associate the problem addiction with something that causes them discomfort or extreme uneasiness. For example, a behavior therapist can teach a patient to associate alcohol with a personal, unpleasant memory.

C. Cognitive-Behavioral Play Therapy

This form of behavior therapy is most commonly and effectively used with children suffering from behavior disorders. When a behavior therapist watches or observes a child play, the behavior therapist is given key insight into how that child reacts to specific situations. For example, behavior therapists can learn what a child is uncomfortable expressing or even unable to express.

Allowing children to play also enables them to feel safe and comfortable. They're free to choose their toys and play at will, allowing behavior therapists the opportunity to glimpse into how that child behaves and reacts. Behavior therapists can also play with a child, so they can gain knowledge and pass it on to parents, enabling parents to implement tactics to have better communication with their children.

D. **System Desensitization**

System desensitization is another form of behavior therapy that is based on the principle of classical conditioning. This type of behavior therapy aims to remove the fear response in reaction a patient has to a phobia. In substitution of the fear, calm or relaxed response to the conditional stimulus begins to gradually develop through counter conditioning.

There are three phases to system desensitization treatment:

1. Physical Treatment: Deep muscle relaxation techniques and breathing exercises are taught. This is an extremely important step because of reciprocal inhibition.
2. Fear Hierarchy: Creating a chart or diagram of what a patient fears least all the way to the most fear-provoking phobia provides a structure for behavior therapy

3. Working the Way Up: Patients working upwards through their fear hierarchy beginning with the fear they are least affected by working there up to the stimulus that provokes the most fear. By moving from stage to stage, the fear patients feel lessens thus making them less prone to being upset or disturbed by it.

By the patient constantly confronting these fears the situations begin to evoke no anxiety. The symptoms or fear that patients feel in reaction to phobias can be successfully treated with system desensitization behavior therapy administered by a professional behavior therapist

Behavioral Therapy

Chapter 3

How Effective is Behavior Therapy?

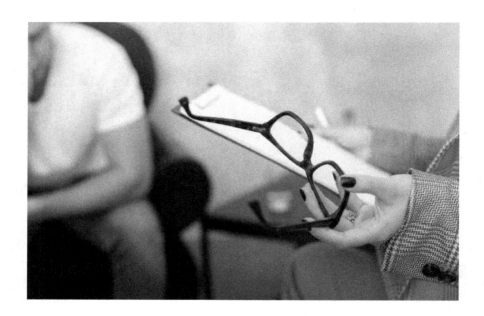

Different types of behavior therapy have been extremely successful in combating different types, and even severities of mental disorders. Not only are different types of behavior therapy effective, but they also address a wide range of

Behavioral Therapy

different mental disorders that a large amount of the population suffers from.

At least 75 percent of patients who go through some form of cognitive behavior therapy benefit positively from treatment to some degree. Although, behavior therapy isn't just dependent on the behavior therapist, the effort the patient puts in as well.

Studies find that behavior therapy techniques are most effective in:

- Depression
- Substance abuse
- Alcoholism
- Paranoia
- Extreme phobias
- Anger issues
- Bulimia and anorexia
- Stress
- Somatoform disorders

Seeking treatment from a behavior therapist can greatly reduce symptoms, if not alleviate them altogether if the proper behavior therapy techniques are used during treatment and supervised by a behavior therapist.

Finding the Right Behavior Therapist

Committing to thoroughly researching a behavior therapist that specializes in the mental disorder you suffer from is hugely important when seeking treatment. If you want to commit to working to rid yourself of your depression or anxiety symptoms, making sure you go online to resources like betterhelp.com and vetting all options should be your first step when trying to find a behavior therapist.

behavior therapist's treatment will involve asking you personal and revealing questions, so not only should you know what practice they are committed to but you should also be sure you are comfortable with them. Comfortability will help you relax and open yourself to treatment, making your recovery easier and the behavior therapist's treatment more effective.

Behavior therapy tends to be short-term, usually lasting between 10 to 20 sessions. Although these sessions with a behavior therapist seem short-lived, their effects are lasting. Committing to behavior therapy can enable you to achieve a level of peace you once thought was impossible.

Treatment can lead to normal reactions, alleviation from depression, elimination of destructive addictions and a permanent curb to fear and anxiety. Certain tasks can now be accomplished without issue.

Finding the right behavior therapist and the right behavior therapy techniques can lead to recovery and the elimination of debilitating symptoms that inhibit you from living your life normally. With commitment, comes recovery.

How to Tell If Your Therapist Uses Cognitive Behavioral Therapy

Cognitive-behavioral therapy is relatively simple, as it's basically changing your thoughts and behavior to feel better emotionally, but in reality, it takes a great deal to be fully trained in how to effectively use this with clients. Although there is no fool-proof way to tell whether your therapist truly is using CBT with you, there are some characteristics to watch for that will make you an informed consumer.

CBT Characteristic 1: Addresses Your Thoughts and Behaviors

A true CBT therapist is going to spend much of your session reviewing the behaviors, thoughts, and emotions that are connected to your main concerns. Often they will use what's called a thought record or, as David Burns, author of the best selling self-help book Feeling Good, calls it, a "Daily Mood Log" to help you capture and then work on your negative thoughts. Almost all therapists will discuss your emotions, at least I hope so, but what sets CBT therapists apart is their additional focus on your thoughts and behaviors. Rather than assuming all your troubles stem from early childhood problems or a traumatic past, CBT therapists will look to your thoughts to determine what to do next. Often your thoughts and behaviors will be automatic or somewhat hidden in nature, and working to draw them out and address them provides substantial relief and great life improvements.

CBT Characteristic 2: Focused and Agenda Driven

Many therapists who don't use CBT often will give advice and be generally supportive, but this can lead to an endless review of your feelings and limited progress. Cognitive-behavioral therapists, although supportive and geared towards your interests as well, differ in that they will set an agenda each session to make sure progress is being made or at least set some structure to make as much movement as possible with each session. This usually involves a short recap of the week, review of homework that was assigned and areas that still need to be addressed, time for practicing techniques, and feedback about the therapy. Although all good therapists will be flexible to some degree depending on what is happening for you at the moment, too much flexibility, combined with the lack of an agenda, often leads to disappointing results.

CBT Characteristic 3: Tracks Your Symptoms

CBT therapists usually monitor your symptoms or the problems that brought you to counseling, in some sort of organized manner. Rather than just asking you how you are feeling, they tend to use standardized tests or scales to keep a close eye on the problems that you are looking for help with. By using such tools, CBT therapists are able to spot trends and quickly react by adapting their therapy to suit your immediate needs. This regular monitoring also allows the therapist and the client both to examine how counseling is going and make decisions about how to proceed.

CBT Characteristic 4: Gives You Helpful Homework

Homework is a hallmark of CBT therapists - and of any good therapists, in my opinion. The research is clear that if you do homework as part of your therapy, you will get better faster and make more progress during your time in counseling. Homework is a requirement of cognitive-behavioral therapy since so much of the counseling is about learning and practicing new skills. Imagine how much more you can do in the week outside of the 50 minutes that you spend with your therapist, and when that work is guided by your experienced therapist, the results are all the more powerful. This being said, not all homework is created equal and an experienced CBT therapist will be able to explain why certain homework is beneficial or needed.

CBT Characteristic 5: Has Received Certification

One clear, but more recent, way to determine if your therapist has some solid CBT skills is to check whether he or she is certified by the Academy of Cognitive Therapy (academyofct.org). This is an organization that was created for just this purpose: to demonstrate clinical competency in cognitive therapy for clients seeking treatment. Becoming certified requires a great deal of training in CBT, letters of recommendation from colleagues, and an extensive description of how you use CBT in your practice, including an audiotape of an actual client session (don't worry, permission must be given by the client).

Seeking therapy is a great way to improve your feelings of anxiety, depression, and stress, and knowing who to see makes it all the easier. If you're looking for time-tested and effective treatment such as cognitive behavioral therapy, the list above can set you in the right direction and help you find a qualified therapist to improve your life.

4.2 Seven Pearls for Effective Cognitive Behavioral Therapy

Research has proven that by identifying our distorted thoughts and beliefs, we can have better control over thoughts, thus better control over our feelings. Having distorted thoughts or beliefs doesn't mean that there is something wrong with us. We all have distorted thoughts and beliefs at different times in our lives. Some examples of distorted thoughts:

Behavioral Therapy

1. Over-Generalizing: At times, we may see things as all-or-nothing. For example, if one thing goes wrong with a project, we may think that the entire project is a failure. Or, if there is one thing that upsets us about a person, we may decide we don't care for that person at all.

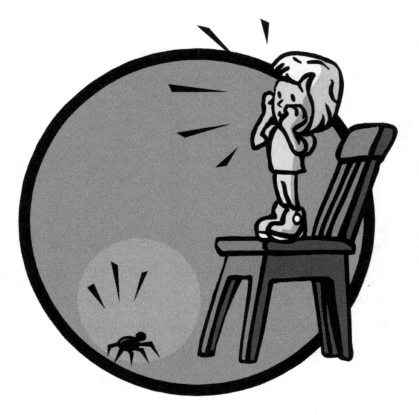

2. Mind Reading: We assume that we know what someone is thinking. We may tell ourselves that

someone thinks we are "stupid" or does not like us even though there is no evidence that supports this thought. This is called mind reading.

3. Catastrophizing: We exaggerate how "awful" something is or imagine the worst possible outcome. Perhaps our boss wants to speak with us and we catastrophize that we are going to be fired. Or, it rains on one of the days of a vacation and we think "this is the worst thing that could have happened".

4. Fortune Telling: We think we know for sure what is going to happen. For example, we tell ourselves, "I know I am not going to get that promotion" or "I won't be able to handle that assignment".

Also, specific behaviors or skills are taught including social skills, assertiveness, organizational skills, and relaxation techniques. These are taught during and between sessions.

Below, are seven pearls that are found helpful

1. Discuss Goals of Treatment

During the initial assessment phase, it is important to collaborate on the goals of treatment. This helps keep the treatment focused and productive. Without goals, therapy can end up focusing on whatever problem is coming up that week and can interfere with the progress of the original presenting problems. Sometimes, the patient may not be able to specifically describe a goal except a vague "I want to be less anxious" or "I want to feel happier". This is fine at the beginning. However, over the first couple of months, you should return to this discussion about goals to see if they can be described in more specific terms.

For example, if someone presents with depression, the goals may include the following: Finding a more fulfilling job, returning to college, exercising three times a week, making two new friends, and stopping the use of marijuana.

2. Start Each Session With An Agenda

Every session should start with an agenda that is discussed collaboratively between the therapist and the patient. Again, this helps to keep the session focused and more effective. The

Behavioral Therapy

agenda should include following up on homework from the previous session, a check-in about the mood and week, bridging or reviewing the topics and progress from the previous session, and

> topics related to discuss in the current session that is related to a specific goal.

3. Discuss Where to Address The Issue

   Most therapy goals will have several components including distorted thoughts, beliefs or behaviors. Thus, during the session, collaboratively decide on which level to address the goals. If you are working on distorted thoughts, it is important to elicit what thoughts or images occur that are leading to distress, such as anxiety, low mood, or blocking a certain behavior. If you are working on certain behaviors such as social skills or relationship issues, it is important to discuss when the skills will be used and how likely it is the skills will be used. Another useful technique for addressing behaviors is role-playing and visualizing which helps to practice the skills and address any blocks or anxieties around the behavior.

4. Use Flashcards

Flashcards can be used to remember the key points of the session or a mantra that may help with certain thoughts or feelings.

5. Stay Focused

At the beginning of treatment, goals for therapy are discussed. Sometimes, the therapy session may head in a direction that is unrelated to any of the goals of treatment. This is appropriate at certain times, but if this is happening every session and for the entire duration, then there can be a limit to the progress of therapy. The structure is important in CBT, but flexibility is also important. This would be a time to collaborate to discuss whether to continue on the current diversion or issue that is being discussed or go back to what was discussed in the agenda.

6. Assign Homework

Towards the end of each session, a collaborative discussion takes place about homework or "action tasks" to perform between sessions. An action task might be to buy a calendar if one of the issues is time management or recording thoughts and images that occur during stressful periods in a notebook to discuss and address at the following session. Always make sure to follow-up on the homework or action task at the next session or it creates the impression that working on problems or goals in between sessions is not a crucial part of getting better.

7. Ask For Feedback

Towards the end of the session, ask what went well during the session, what could have gone better, and what the main take-away messages are. This helps to build the alliance, improve future sessions, and maximize progress.

Cognitive-behavioral therapy is an extremely effective form of therapy, either with or without medications and is an excellent way to practice psychiatry.

Behavioral Therapy

CPSIA information can be obtained
at www.ICGtesting.com
Printed in the USA
BVHW041353200421
605393BV00001B/178